Walking, Fitness, You

Step Into a Walking Routine, Everything You Need to Know

By Ryder Management Inc.

Epitaph

"Walking with a friend in the dark is better than walking alone in the light."

Helen Keller

"Walking is a Man's best medicine."

Hippocrates

.

Table of Contents

Introduction

Did you know that walking is the number one participation sport on the planet? Although there are countless physical activities to choose from, walking is reported to have the lowest dropout rate out of all of them. In addition, walking can be either a solo event, shared with a walking group, or shared with only your best friend.

Walking is easy to do. It does not require any special skill, advanced training or conditioning. It also does not require any special equipment or clothing. All you really need to get started is a good pair of walking shoes, some comfortable clothing, a water bottle and perhaps a pedometer to count and track your steps.

Walking is a low risk activity and is very easy to start. Walking will help keep you fit and reduce your risk of serious diseases such as heart disease, diabetes, obesity, stroke and depression to name just a few.

According to a study by the Centre for Disease Control (CDC), less than one-half of Americans are engaged in the minimum-recommended 150 minutes per week of physical activity. This amount (150 minutes per week) can be broken down into 30 minutes for five days each week.

This ebook is written for those of you living a relatively inactive life, regardless of how the inactivity began. The purpose of this book is to inspire and encourage you to begin your own individual walking routine. The benefits you will gain out of a regular routine of daily walks will surely make those who love you very proud of you. In addition, your self-esteem will increase as well as your natural beauty.

This book was written to provide you with all the information, and then some, regarding getting started in a regular walking routine.

Benefits of Walking

The list of walking benefits is long. In fact, research into the health benefits of walking continue to increase as new benefits are discovered on a daily basis. Some of the health benefits of walking include:

Walking eases back pain.

Walking reduces your waist line.

Walking lowers blood pressure.

Walking reduces levels of bad cholesterol (LDL).

Walking increases the level of HDL (good cholesterol).

Walking reduces heart attack risk.

Walking improves the health of your heart and lungs.

Walking reduces the risk of Type 2 diabetes.

Walking reduces and lessens stress and anxiety.

Walking is easy on your joints.

Walking reduces the appetite.

Walking improves muscle tone, muscle strength and muscle endurance.

Walking enhances stamina and energy.

Walking reduces heart attack risk and the risk of heart disease.

Walking reduces the risk of certain types of cancer.

Walking reduces the risk of chronic disease.

Walking slows down osteoporosis bone loss.

Walking improves balance and coordination.

Walking can be done anytime, including holidays, business travel, morning noon and night.

Walking increases aerobic capacity.

Walking strengthens your heart.

Walking lowers the risk of illness.

Walking keeps your weight in check and can help you to lose weight.

Walking improves your sleep and regulates your sleeping cycle.

Walking helps prevent dementia.

Walking can strengthen your memory.

Walking increases your mood.

Walking can boost your self-esteem.

Walking boosts immune function.

Walking allows you to gather your thoughts.

Walking gives you time to think.

Walking can be a form of meditation.

Walking contributes to reduced body fat.

Walking improves glycemic control, particularly after eating meals.

Walking helps you to live longer.

Walking can reduce pain.

Walking can help prevent falls in seniors.

Walking gets you out of the house.

Walking on a regular basis will get you in shape.

Walking can help you meet new friends.

Walking will make your skin glow.

Walking will make you feel good and therefore, look good.

Walking is a good form of transportation.

Walking is good for the environment.

Walking slows the aging process.

Walking is all-inclusive.

Fitness Basics

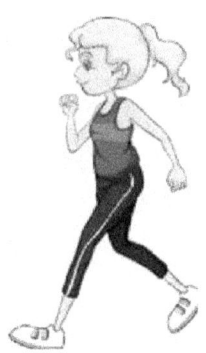

Starting any fitness program is one of the most important and best things you can do for your health. As itemized in the previous chapter, the list of benefits associated with walking continues to grow each day. Regardless of your age, sex or physical ability, walking can reduce your risk of chronic disease, boost your self-esteem and help you lose or control your weight.

The Department of Health and Human Services recommends that healthy individuals include a form of aerobic exercise and strength training into their fitness plans. More specifically, they recommend at least 150 minutes of moderate aerobic activity each week. Alternatively, you can include 75 minutes of vigorous aerobic activity to achieve the same results. In other words, vigorous aerobic activity would entail a brisk power walk on a regular basis.

Although starting a fitness program is an important decision, it should not be an overwhelming one. By planning carefully and starting slowly by pacing yourself, you can make fitness a daily habit that will reap you a lifetime of positive benefits.

The 4-1-1 on Stretching

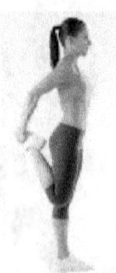

Quad Stretch

Stretching is an important and powerful part of any exercise program, including walking. Most aerobic and strength training exercises, such as walking, inherently cause muscles to contract and tighten, causing sore and aching muscles. Stretching your muscles after your walking routine is important to prevent them from becoming stiff and sore.

Stretching your muscles after your walk will help improve the range of motion in your joints, increase blood circulation and help to prevent sore muscles.

As in most things, it is necessary to know and become familiar with certain rules so that you gain the most from your new walking routine. To begin with, it is important to remember to never stretch cold muscles. The best time to stretch your muscles is after your walk or during your walk, once you have warmed up. However, if you know you have problem areas in your body, these areas can be stretched prior to beginning your walk.

The best warm-up exercise for your walk is to start with a five (5) minute walking warm-up. Start by walking at a medium pace and then slowly increase your pace so that by the end of the five minutes, you can easily begin your walking routine by continuing into it.

Stretching your muscles after you exercise can help you to increase the range of motion in your joints. Remember to begin your stretch slowly and hold it gently. Only stretch to the point of feeling a gentle pull, but never to the point of pain. If you do feel pain, you have gone too far. Forget "No Pain No Gain"; it does not apply to us in our walking routine.

When you are stretching, keep it gentle; breathe freely while holding your stretch; hold each stretch for 20 to 30 seconds, and then release. If you have any problems with a stretch, hold for a lesser time and then repeat the stretch. To begin, each stretch should be done once if holding for thirty seconds, or twice if holding for a count of 15 seconds. Seniors will benefit by working up to a count of 60 seconds per stretch.

The Best Post Walking Leg Stretches

Quad stretch:

Pictured above, you may want to use a wall, fence or post to help with balance and stability. Since the quadriceps muscles are used in walking, it is necessary to stretch these muscles after your walk to prevent soreness. To begin, stand erect and bend your knee behind you so that you can grasp your foot from behind and hold your heel against your butt. Hold this position for 15-30 seconds before releasing your foot. Stand on both feet and then repeat this stretch with your opposite foot.

Hip flexor stretch:

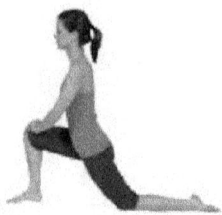

To stretch the right hip flexors, kneel on your right knee and put your left foot in front of you. Your left hip and knee should be about 90 degrees. If you find this position, pictured above, uncomfortable, consider putting a cushion on the floor, under your knee. Keep your chest up and be sure not to bend forward at the hips. Hold this position for 15-30 seconds and then stand on both feet before switching to your left hip flexors. Repeat.

Hamstring stretch:

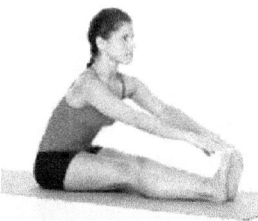

Hamstrings are very strong muscles and may take months of stretching to get them to a reasonably flexible level. Therefore, please do not expect any quick results.

To begin stretching your hammies, sit on the floor with your legs straight in front of you. Sit up straight and breathe in. Breathe out and bend at your hips reaching forward to touch your toes. Make sure that your toes are pointing up. Hold this forward stretch for 15-30 seconds as you feel the stretch in your hamstrings. Return to sitting up straight. Repeat this exercise.

Calf stretch:

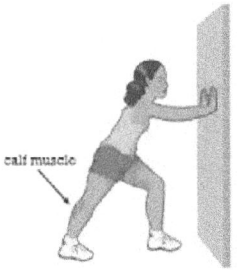

calf muscle

The calf muscle actually consists of two muscles: the gastrocnemius and the deeper muscle called the soleus. Both of these insert into the Achilles tendon located at the back of your ankle. Since the gastrocnemius originates from above your knee, in order to stretch it, the knee must be fully extended. Since the soleus muscle originates below the knee, the knee need not be extended in order to stretch this muscle.

Stand away from the wall and put your right foot behind you ensuring your toes are facing the wall. Keeping your heel on the ground, lean forward with your right knee straight and hold this position for 30 seconds. Return to standing position and repeat with your left leg.

Stand away from the wall and put your right foot behind you ensuring your toes are facing the wall. Lean forward at the ankle while bending your right knee, keeping your heel on the ground. Hold this position for 30 seconds. Return to standing position and repeat with your left leg.

Butterfly/groin stretch:

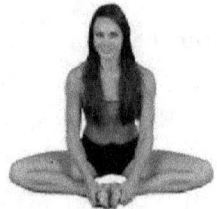

Sit on the floor with your knees bent and your feet pulled together so that your legs are in the butterfly position, pictured above. Put your hands around your ankles. Keeping your spine straight and your butt pressed into the floor and slowly bend forward at the waist. Using your elbows, carefully press them against your knees, gently pushing them apart. It is important not to round your back. Hold this position for 15-30 seconds before relaxing. Repeat up to three times.

Key Walking Tips

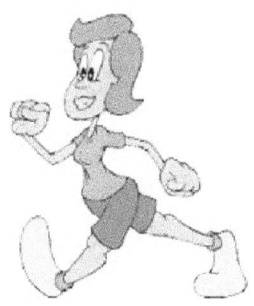

In order to get the most out of walking, remember that good posture is crucial. Practice good posture while you are walking by remembering to keep your head up while looking straight ahead (although it is important to look down occasionally in order to avoid any sudden obstacle that can otherwise trip you). It is important to also keep your spine straight and your stride should be no more than up to a comfortable 30 inches. Your arms and shoulders should be loose while you take deep regular breaths. Never hold your breath.

To get the most out of your walk, walk and don't run. Remember to keep a brisk pace, but not a fast one. Shortly after you begin walking, you should be able to determine a correct pace for yourself. If you find yourself running out of breath, slow your pace down because you are walking too fast. You should be able to carry on a comfortable conversation as you walk at a "brisk" pace.

Your stride should be long and smooth and the motion in your stride should be relatively effortless. Your arms should be swinging at your side as they provide balance.

The phrase "If it feels good, do it" applies to walking. In addition, the opposite of this phrase is also true. If you find yourself with sore muscles, consider stretching longer or increasing the number of stretches you do that are specific to the area on your body that is sore.

A Quick Look at Common Walking Mistakes

There is a proper way to walk and walking the right way can help give you more enjoyment, better health, fitness and even a better attitude. Avoiding certain walking mistakes can also assist you with walking faster and more smoothly. Walking the wrong way can lead to wasted effort and even injury. Therefore, the following are common walking mistakes to avoid.

Overstriding:

When walkers try to walk faster, their first inclination is to increase their stride by reaching further with their forward foot. If you are attempting to increase your walking speed, concentrate on taking shorter and quicker steps. This increases the number of steps per second.

Wearing the wrong shoes:

Not all shoes are made for walking. Your walking shoes should be lightweight and flexible. If your shoes have soles that won't bend easily, they are too stiff and can cause knee and/or foot problems in the long run. Walking shoes should be replaced every 500 miles or six months when used regularly. The cushioning and support in your walking shoes do degrade over time. Your walking shoes should also be larger than your dress shoes if you engage in walking for exercise for 30 minutes or more. The reason for this is to accommodate your feet when they swell.

Not using your arms:

Keeping your arms stiff at your side will slow you down. By bending your arms and letting them swing naturally will add power and speed to your walk and help you obtain the maximum benefits from it.

Incorrect posture including walking with your head down or leaning forward:

Good posture, chin up and parallel to the ground will allow you to breathe better and will help to prevent any potential problems with your back, neck and shoulders. By strengthening your abdominal muscles through sit-ups has the added benefit of helping you to hold yourself straighter during your walk. Therefore, you are encouraged to think this over and start squeezing in sit-ups, even if you only do five at a time to start.

Wearing the wrong clothes:

Clothing mistakes include wearing too much or not enough, depending on the weather. In addition, wearing dark clothing at night is another common mistake to avoid. For comfort when walking, remember to dress in layers.

Becoming dehydrated:

In order to stay hydrated, it is important to drink a glass of water every hour throughout each day. In addition, ten minutes prior to your walk, drink a glass of water. Remember to bring your water bottle on your walk as it is recommended to drink a cup of water every 20 minutes.

Over doing it:

If you feel that you are losing your enthusiasm for waking, you may have been over doing it. If you feel tired and irritable with aches and pains, you have definitely overextended yourself. If any of these situations apply to you, it is important that you take a break from your walking routine. The best thing for you to do is to rest and catch up on your sleep.

The above was just a quick overview of common walking mistakes for you to remember and hopefully think about and keep in mind.

Walking Gear

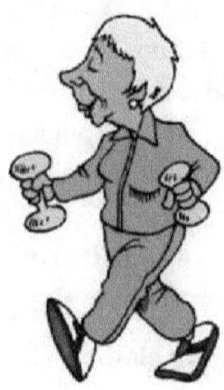

Although walking only really involves putting one foot in front of the other, there are a number of things that can increase your walking enjoyment.

The most important consideration with your walking routine is choosing your walking footwear. In this regard, ensure that your footwear is as comfortable as possible, according to you. This means that you can make do with the footwear you presently have, but make sure to choose the most comfortable pair of walking shoes you presently own.

When you are able to shop for a new pair of walking shoes, make sure that the shoes have proper arch support, according to what's right for your individual feet. The arch should not be stiff. Ensuring arch flexibility will allow each foot to easily roll from heel to toe when stepping. A stiff shoe or one not broken in will invariably cause pain by putting undue stress on each foot. Another important factor with regards to walking shoes is their flexibility.

Once you start feeling and noticing the benefits of your uninterrupted daily walking routine, you may want to consider adding to your walking gear. In this regard, consider the following:

Shoes: The choice and decision of type of shoes is a personal one. If you choose to give the decision to others, you may find yourself buying a large selection of shoes that don't really work for you.

Socks: Rather than the common cotton sock, consider socks made of hemp or any similar absorbent of liquid compounds including sweat.

Clothing: Wearing what is comfortable to you is of utmost importance; do consider layering your walking gear. This includes looser fitting tops over top of tighter shirts such as sleeveless camisoles.

Sport Bras: Women of all sizes struggle to be comfortable while out walking. The problem we encounter when it comes to bras and walking include chafing, slipping straps, proper support and using the right bra. To this end, we have devoted a chapter to this important factor.

Water Bottles: Please don't forget to keep hydrated. The easiest way to ensure you are not dehydrated is to always carry a water bottle with you. While out walking, there are many new and nifty ways to carry your filtered water such as those that strap onto your back. Regardless of how you choose to sport your water, the most important thing to remember is – not to forget to bring your water on your walk.

Pedometers: The most basic pedometer is an electronic device that counts your steps. In order to obtain a good reading, these devices must be adjusted to your stride length. The more current models now come with a variety of new features. The most sophisticated versions even include a GPS system that can accurately calculate speed and distance based on satellite readings, and of course are able to determine your exact where about.

A Personal Stereo, IPod or MP3 Player: When walking alone, a music device can be make your routine that much more enjoyable. Not only can the music motivate and inspire you, it can energize your workout while helping to pass the time by creating a very enjoyable distraction.

Walking Gait and Walking Shoes

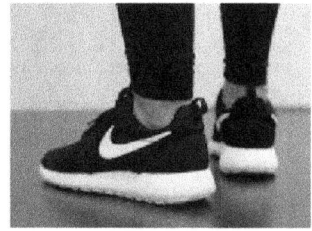

Shoes are the single most important piece of walking equipment and can make the difference between an enjoyable walk and an uncomfortable, painful walk. It is important to use a good pair of walking shoes that provide both support and comfort to all parts of your feet. Your walking shoes should provide enough toe room to enable you to wiggle your toes yet provide firm heel support. The sole of your walking shoes should be cushioned and flexible in order to aid in your walking gait and to also absorb shock. Your walking shoes should be lightweight and made of breathable material, preferably leather or fabric that allows perspiration to dissipate.

Walking gait:

Walking gait is defined by Dictionary.com as the manner of walking, stepping or running. Your walking gait is unique to you but is important in choosing your walking shoes.

By examining the bottom of your walking shoes, a great deal can be learned about your walking gait or manner in which you walk. Depending on wear your shoe is worn sheds light on your walking gait. An expert athletic shoe specialist that is selling you brand new walking shoes should take this into account along with watching you walk when determining the best kind of footwear based on this information.

Overpronation:

Overpronation is defined as excessive inward or medial movement; a rolling inwards of your foot. Overpronators have a stride in which their ankle rolls too much inward with each step. This excessive roll will tend to cause strain to the ankle, knee and shins. Motion control shoes will help Overpronators by having a much stiffer heel and medial support that helps prevent the foot from rolling too far inward. If your gait is normal, you do not need motion control shoes.

Supination (Under-pronation):

Supination is the opposite of Overpronation. Supination is defined as an insufficient inward roll of the foot after landing. This condition places undue stress on the foot and knee. Supinators should do extra stretching for the calves, hamstrings and quads.

Although self-diagnosis is one thing, it is important to consult a live fitness specialist to help analyze your gait and help you purchase a shoe that is unique to you.

Pedometers

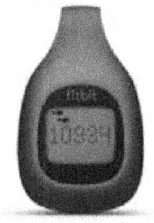

Walking as a highly effective fitness program has evolved over the last few years. As a result, the choice in pedometer style and options has also greatly expanded. A pedometer is an electronic device that, in its simplest form, tracks the number of steps you make. A pedometer senses your body motion and through this, is able to count your footsteps. This footstep count is then converted into distance using the length of your average stride. Incorporating a pedometer into your walking program can act as a great motivator and can be worn all day, every day or just when you go out for your fitness walk.

According to a study by Harvard Alumni, it reported that walking an average of 6,000 steps per day produced the greatest reduction in death rates. The amount of 6,000 steps per day, for most people, translates into walking about an hour every day. By wearing your pedometer all day, you can determine how close you are to achieving the 6,000 accumulated steps per day.

The average accumulated steps most people achieve in a day, without any additional exercise devoted to walking, has been logged at 3,000 steps per day. It should be kept in mind that the number of steps required in a day to burn off extra calories for weight loss is 10,000 steps per day.

The number and sophistication of available options on the most current pedometers today is nothing short of amazing.

A leading pedometer manufacturer is the maker of the FitBit Zip, pictured above. This model can be worn indiscreetly on your belt, pocket or even your bra. This model, basic in its class, can track steps, distance and calories burned, which seems to be the basic feature in all the basic pedometers on the market today.

In addition, the FitBit Zip pedometer syncs automatically to your computer or with Bluetooth to select smartphones and tablets. It also includes options such as setting fitness goals, fitness progress and the ability of earning and displaying badges. Most pedometers on the market today also include a stopwatch, time/date feature as well as an alarm clock too. The alarm can be set to wake you up and these models also have the ability to monitor how long and how well you sleep.

Other pedometer models, such as the Fitness Paal by Quorum International, come equipped with an attack alarm that is loud enough to wake the neighborhood.

Due to the vast selection of options available with any pedometer, it is necessary to do your homework and shop around in order that you get the best bang for your buck.

The Accuracy of the Various Pedometer Mechanisms

A question most people ask regarding pedometers is with respect to their accuracy. The accuracy of a pedometer depends on the type and model of the device. Generally, the accuracy of an acceptable pedometer should have an error rate of 10% or less.

Although all pedometers count steps, they use different methods or mechanisms of accomplishing this.

There are basically three types of pedometers that can be categorized according to its mechanism that control it and these include the accelerometer, coiled spring mechanism and the hairspring mechanism. The coiled spring and hairspring mechanisms are both spring-load models.

The least accurate method that counts steps is the hairspring mechanism and is the model that is usually given away or included in free health promotions. The hairspring model is also the least expensive and offers the least amount of features. As time passes, these models also become less accurate due to the spring losing elasticity over time with use.

The spring on the coil model has less probability of loosening as time passes and therefore has a longer life compared to the hairspring models. The newer of these models are electronic and also come with additional features that usually include a clock, number of calories burned, an accumulation log that can report weekly and monthly accumulated activity. These coiled spring models are usually attached to your belt or waistband byway of a clip. In order to get an accurate reading from this type of pedometer, they must remain in the vertical position. This vertical position can be a problem when used by someone who is overweight and carrying extra abdominal baggage because when these models are tilted forward, which is a common occurrence when the excess abdominal fat pushes the waist attached spring loaded pedometer forward. Tilt in a spring-levered pedometer can throw off their accuracy by as much as 20% at slow speeds and by an astounding 60% at high speeds.

The most accurate and consequently the more costly type of pedometer available is the accelerometer, also known as piezoelectric pedometer. This type is also more durable and has no moving parts that can wear out. This type uses the technology of two or three axis microelectromechanical system (MEMS). Piezoelectric pedometers also tend to be more sensitive than spring levered at slow speeds and therefore are suited for those individuals that tend to walk more slowly. It should also be pointed out that piezoelectric or accelerometer devices are not position dependent.

Measuring distance and calories

All pedometers do not measure distance or calories burned with an acceptable rate of accuracy. In fact, distance is usually out by an error rate exceeding 10% and calories burned usually have an error rate exceeding 30% in all models. Due to these unacceptable error rates to which pedometers are prone, it is advisable to use a simple pedometer that measures only steps with an accuracy rate greater than 90% (or conversely, an error rate of less than 10%).

Testing your pedometer

Your pedometer should be worn on your waist and in a straight line that is measured from the middle of your knee. You can place your pedometer on either side of your body, above either your left or right knee.

In order to determine the accuracy of the pedometer you choose to use, set your pedometer to zero and then walk and count out exactly 100 steps. Once you have walked exactly 100 counted steps, compare to the reading on your pedometer. Remember that the pedometer is accurate if the error is within 10% of your counted steps. In other words, if your pedometer reads anywhere between 90 to 110 steps, it can be considered accurate.

Although a number of factors can affect the accuracy of a pedometer, the two most important ones are where you wear it and your stride length. As already mentioned the most accurate pedometer is the ones with an accelerometer mechanism and these ones can be worn clipped to your bra, shoe or even carried in your pocket as these ones are not affected by positioning.

Pedometers do require you to enter your stride length when setting up your pedometer for the first time. In this regard, follow the instructions that come with your pedometer carefully because stride length is very important to any pedometer's accuracy.

If the error rate of your pedometer is greater than 10% (it reads either greater than 110 steps or less than 90 steps), give it another chance by repositioning it on your body. You can try switching sides or positioning and repeating the exercise of 100 steps. Don't forget to reset your pedometer to zero when you are retesting it. If after many repeated tests, if the error rate is still greater than 10%, do consider exchanging your model at the place where you purchased it.

When shopping for a pedometer, Amazon alone has over 21,000 models to choose from. The advantage with beginning your shopping at Amazon is that the posted reviews from other buyers can be an invaluable source of information for you PLUS you are able to avoid any salesperson trying to sell you a more expensive model that supposedly includes all the bells and whistles. As discussed above, all you really need is accuracy in the ability to count your steps, period.

Sport Bras

Women of all sizes have a unique issue with being comfortable while walking. Using the right bra, such as a sports bra, is critical in the elimination of problems that ordinary bras can cause when walking.

Problems caused by the average bra when walking:

In order to understand how a sports bra can increase your walking enjoyment, problems associated with wearing an ordinary bra when walking are discussed below and include:

Slipping bra straps that fall off your shoulders become very annoying especially while in motion. Also, if you are carrying a backpack, a problem with the straps rubbing can be compounded because of the backpack. Most sport bras today offer racer-back or T-back designs that prevent the straps from slipping off your shoulders.

Sometimes motion can cause bra hooks to become unhooked, causing an embarrassing episode. Racer-back bras are available without hooks and simply slide over your head.

Cotton and all cotton bras turn into sweat mops if you are prone to sweat when walking. Since most bras are made of cotton, it is necessary to look for sport bras that can offer sweat control.

When the warm weather arrives, where there is sweat and motion, there is chafing. Chafing is defined by the online dictionary Encarta as soreness or wear caused by rubbing.

Since most ordinary bras scream "underwear" if worn alone, in most instances you are not able to remove your outer shirt in public when wearing an average bra underneath. This can be quite problematic on hot days if you become very hot and start to overheat. In these instances, being able to wear a sports bra is a godsend.

The bra and bra style to choose depends on which problems you need to solve. The worst problem of all is unique to ladies with larger cup sizes and is that of support. Since gravity will do wreck its own havoc, big breasted women certainly require bras offering good support in order to prevent black eyes from their otherwise unsupported flapping "girls".

For ladies with smaller cup sizes, the average spandex mixed sports bra can produce very unflattering flattened results. Therefore, a trade-off between comfort and appearance is necessary.

Closing Remarks

Making a personal commitment to sticking to your walking routine is of utmost importance to your health and well-being. Make a personal decision to stick to your walking routine by setting aside time each day or at least for five times every week. Consider using your daily planner by scheduling in time to walk each day, the same way you do when making any appointment of great importance. By making exercise a priority, just like work and family obligations, can greatly increase the value of everyday life for you.

Consider going back and revisiting the number of benefits associated with walking, two of which are reduced stress and increased moods.

In order to get the most out of life, it is important to do your best to balance your life as best as you can. This includes eating properly, setting aside time for yourself including exercising, setting aside time for your family and leaving work at the office whether the office is at home or outside of your home.

Remember if you don't have your health, you won't be able to enjoy your life.

I sincerely hope that this book has provided value to you. If you enjoyed this book, please tell others, if not, please tell us.

info@RyderManagement.ca

.

References and Resources

Lee IM, Paffenbarger RS Jr. "Associations of light, moderate, and vigorous intensity physical activity with longevity. The Harvard Alumni Health Study." Am J Epidemiol. 2000 Feb 1;151(3):293-9.

Map My Walk – an online site for finding a walking club anywhere in the world. http://www.mapmywalk.com

Best Rated Walking Shoes for Women in 2015: http://www.the-fitness-walking-guide.com/womens-walking-shoes.html

Nordic Walking Meetups: http://nordic-walking.meetup.com/

Amazon's Top Rated Pedometers: http://www.amazon.com/gp/top-rated/hpc/219599011

Lumo Lift: http://www.amazon.com/s/ref=nb_sb_noss?url=search-alias%3Daps&field-keywords=lumo+lift

About the Author

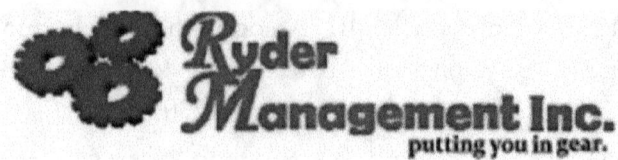

Ryder Management Inc. (Rydermgt or RMI) is a Canadian Controlled Private Corporation (CCPC) based in London, ON Canada. As an "umbrella" organization, *Rydermgt* brings together a group of authors whom are professionals in their respective fields and are writing with the primary goal of providing books that educate, comfort and offer assurance that natural health remedies do exist and are an effective and safe way to regain, obtain and maintain our health.

Please see Ryder Management Inc's author page at Amazon: http://www.amazon.com/Ryder-Management-Inc/e/B00ICGMCRS

for a list of over 25 books published by Ryder Management Inc.